Coding Solutions

EVALUATION AND MANAGEMENT SERVICES

2025 Edition

Improve Documentation - Code Intelligently - Minimize Audit Risk

Piyush N. Sheth, MD, FACS, DABS

ISBN: 978-0-9969672-9-7

International Classification of Diseases (ICD)

ICD is copyright by the World Health Organization. ICD10 codes used in this book were adapted from the U.S. modification (ICD10-CM) available on the CMS website as tabular and index pdf files. Please refer to the official ICD10-CM publication to confirm codes.

Current Procedural Terminology (CPT®)

CPT codes, descriptions and other data are copyright American Medical Association. All rights reserved. CPT is a registered trademark of the American Medical Association (AMA). Please refer to the official CPT code set from the AMA to confirm codes.

Resource Based Relative Value Scale (RBRVS)

Developed by Harvard University and maintained by CMS (Centers for Medicare & Medicaid Services). This book uses current work RVUs (relative value units) that were available at the time of publication.

Disclaimer of Warranties and Liabilities

This book is provided "as is" without warranty of any kind, either expressed or implied. It is solely meant to be a reference for Evaluation and Management Services coding and the user is encouraged to confirm codes prior to submission from official sources. This book is not meant to be all inclusive. Piyush N. Sheth, MD, bears no liability for any results or consequences that may arise from the use of this book.

Disclosures

Piyush N. Sheth, MD, is an employed physician. This book is an independent work and is wholly owned by Piyush N. Sheth, MD. All rights reserved.

Piyush N. Sheth, MD, has accepted no endorsements or financial benefits from any third party in the publishing of this book.

CONTENTS

PAGE

PREFACE

Vita Brevis, Ars Longa.

Life is short, the art of medicine is long, opportunity fleeting, experience perilous, and judgement difficult.

David B. Adams, MD, FACS, Medical University of South Carolina, Charleston

This book is intended for Healthcare Providers (physicians, APP's, etc.) and Professional Medical Coders. It provides a streamlined process for Evaluation and Management Services medical coding and documentation to achieve efficiency and accuracy in medical billing.

THE PROBLEM

The **ICD-10-CM (International Classification of Diseases, version 10, Clinical Modification) code set** was adopted in the U.S. on October 1, 2015 and is updated annually by Medicare. The Optum360® ICD-10-CM Expert for Physicians is **approximately 1,300 pages and contains about 74,000 codes** (excluding the Coding Guidelines and Appendices).

The **AMA CPT® (Current Procedural Terminology) Professional Edition** is updated annually and contains over **11,000 codes within its 1,300 pages.** Due to years of additions, deletions, and revisions, some codes are out of sequence making it inherently inefficient.

The **Federal Register Annual Final Rules for Medicare and Medicaid Programs are over 1,000 pages** and includes Payment Policies Under the Physician Fee Schedule and Other Changes to Part B Payment and Coverage Policies, Medicare Shared Savings Program Requirements, Medicare Advantage, Medicare and Medicaid Provider and Supplier Enrollment Policies, and Basic Health Program.

The **Medicare Claims Processing Manual – Chapter 12 – Physicians and NPP's is almost 200 pages.**

The **Omnibus Budget Reconciliation Act of 1989** enacted the Medicare Physician Fee Schedule. It provides for the **RVUs (Relative Value Units)** that value physician services. **The Balanced Budget Act of 1997** permits Congress to determine the conversion factor that translates RVU's into payment values.

Electronic Medical Record's (EMR) were designed to provide ease in documentation, minimize medical errors, and allow ubiquitous access to medical records. Today, we recognize that EMRs are complex, tedious to use, propagate medical errors, do not allow facile sharing of medical information across different vendor systems, and allow for the effortless commission of fraud (either intentional or unintentional). ***The dictum "if it's not documented, you didn't do it" no longer holds true; EMRs allow you to easily "document what you didn't do."*** Furthermore, they have poorly designed search algorithms for both ICD and CPT codes.

The result: *complexity, inefficiency, frustration, and errors.*

THE SOLUTION

Develop an affordable, concise, portable, and easy to use reference for Evaluation and Management coding, and include numerous other efficiency guides pertaining to documentation, coding, and best practices.

Medicare has set the standard: ***the physician is responsible for the proper documentation and use of codes when submitting claims.*** Improper documentation and coding leads to denied claims, wasted resources when resubmitting claims, lost revenue from writing off claims if they are perceived as non-payable, and ultimately allegations of fraud with resultant audits and penalties. All healthcare providers and coders are encouraged to be cognizant of this.

I hope you find this book to be an indispensable addition to your coding library.

Piyush N. Sheth

ONLINE REFERENCES

1. Federal Register Final Rule Medicare and Medicaid Programs; CY 2024 Payment Policies Under the Physician Fee Schedule and Other Changes to Part B Payment and Coverage Policies; Medicare Shared Savings Program Requirements; Medicare Advantage; Medicare and Medicaid Provider and Supplier Enrollment Policies; and Basic Health Program – (12/09/2024) 1,348 pages
   https://www.federalregister.gov/documents/2024/12/09/2024-25382/medicare-and-medicaid-programs-cy-2025-payment-policies-under-the-physician-fee-schedule-and-other
2. Medicare Claims Processing Manual – Chapter 12 – Physicians and NPPs – 192 pages
   https://www.cms.gov/Regulations-and-Guidance/Guidance/Manuals/Downloads/clm104c12.pdf
3. Medicare Physician Fee Schedule Lookup:
   https://www.cms.gov/apps/physician-fee-schedule/license-agreement.aspx
4. CPT® Evaluation and Management (E/M) Office or Other Outpatient Code and Guideline Changes, 01/01/2021 – 28 pages
   https://www.ama-assn.org/system/files/2019-06/cpt-office-prolonged-svs-code-changes.pdf
5. CPT® Evaluation and Management (E/M) Hospital Code and Guideline Changes, 01//01/2023, 42 pages
   https://www.ama-assn.org/system/files/2023-e-m-descriptors-guidelines.pdf

ABBREVIATIONS

AMA	American Medical Association
CF	Conversion Factor
CMS	Centers for Medicare and Medicaid Services (a.k.a. Medicare)
CPT	Common Procedural Terminology (developed by the AMA)
E/M	Evaluation and Management
EMR / EHR	Electronic Medical Record / Electronic Health Record
GPCI	Geographic Practice Cost Index
HCFA	Healthcare Finance Administration (changed to CMS on June 14, 2001)
HCPCS	Healthcare Common Procedure Coding System (Level I codes are CPT codes)
HHS	Health and Human Services
HIPAA	Health Insurance Portability and Accountability Act
HPI	History of Present Illness
ICD	International Classification of Diseases
MDM	Medical Decision Making
NCCI	National Correct Coding Initiative
NPP	Non-physician practitioner (e.g., Nurse Practitioner)
OIG	Office of the Inspector General
ONC	The Office of the National Coordinator for Health Information Technology
PFSH	Past, Family and Social History
POS	Place of Service
QHP	Qualified Healthcare Professional – An individual qualified to perform a professional service within his/her scope of practice by education, training, licensure/regulation and facility privileging.
RBRVS	Resource Based Relative Value Scale
ROS	Review of Systems
RVU	Relative Value Unit
WHO	World Health Organization

HISTORICAL TIMELINE OF CODING AND DOCUMENTATION

YEAR	EVENT
1847	American Medical Association (AMA) formed.
1872	Nomenclature of Diseases, AMA.
1893	International List of Causes of Death, International Statistical Institute.
1909	ICD-1 (International Classification of Disease, version 1) introduced.
1919	Standard Nomenclature of Diseases and Pathological Conditions, Injuries, and Poisonings for the United States, US Census Bureau.
1946	ICD delegated to the World Health Organization by the United Nations.
1961	Standard Nomenclature of Diseases and Operations (SNDO), Final edition.
1965	Inception of Medicare and Medicaid Programs by President Lyndon B. Johnson.
1966	CPT-1 (Current Procedural Terminology) introduced, AMA.
1977	The Healthcare Financing Administration (HCFA) was formed.
1979	ICD-9-CM implemented [13,000 codes].
1983	HCFA adopts CPT as Level 1 HCPCS.
1988	American Academy of Professional Coders (AAPC) founded.
1988	Resource-Based Relative Value Scale (RBRVS) created at Harvard University.
1989	Omnibus Budget Reconciliation Act.
1992	Medicare implements RBRVS and the Physician Fee Schedule.
1995	1995 Evaluation/Management Documentation guidelines implemented.
1996	Health Insurance Portability and Accountability Act (HIPAA).
1997	1997 Evaluation/Management Documentation guidelines implemented.
2001	HCFA renamed as the Centers for Medicare and Medicaid Services (CMS).
2015	ICD-10-CM implemented [68,000 codes].
2021	Evaluation/Management Documentation and Coding Guidelines Revised for Office / Outpatient Services, "Patients over Paperwork" initiative by CMS and AMA.
2023	Evaluation/Management Documentation and Coding Guidelines Revised for Hospital Inpatient Services, AMA.
2024	Revision of Definitions of Shared / Split services and Time Based coding.

RBRVS AND RVU's

William Hsiao and a team of researchers at Harvard University developed the RBRVS (Resource-Based Relative Value Scale) in 1988. It is based on a 'relative value' of a service and the resources it consumes. There are three components: physician work, practice expense, and malpractice expense. Payment for a service is determined by multiplying the Relative Value Unit (RVU) of the service with the GPCI (Geographic Practice Cost Index) for the CMS locality and by the Medicare conversion factor. President George H. W. Bush signed into law the Omnibus Budget Reconciliation Act of 1989 that switched Medicare to a RBRVS payment system. CMS implemented the RBRVS Physician Fee Schedule on January 1, 1992. Many third-party payers utilize variations of the Medicare RBRVS.

NOTA BENE

RBRVS is important for employed physician models that reimburse based on work RVU productivity.

Physician Work RVU (wRVU) – It includes physician time, mental effort, technical skill, physical effort, judgment, stress and an amortization of the physician's education. The AMA's RUC (Relative Value Scale Update Committee) provides input to CMS regarding the physician wRVU.

Practice Expense RVU (PE RVU) – Some services have two PE RVUs: one for procedures performed in a facility (hospital, ambulatory surgery center, etc.) and one for procedures performed at non-facility sites (e.g., physician's office).

Malpractice Expense (MP RVU) – This is based on malpractice premium data. It is updated at least every 5 years by CMS.

Geographic Practice Cost Index (GPCI) – This reflects the relative costs associated with providing services in a specific Medicare locality compared to national average relative costs. The Cost of Living GPCI applies to wRVUs. The Practice Cost GPCI applies to PE RVUs. The Professional Liability Insurance Cost GPCI applies to MP RVUs.

Medicare Conversion Factor (CF) – This is a national value updated by Congress yearly that converts RVUs into payment amounts as specified by the Balanced Budget Act of 1997.

Year	*2011*	*2012*	*2013*	*2014*	*2015*	*2016*	*2017*	*2018*	*2019*	*2020*	*2021*	*2022*
Conversion Factor	33.98	34.04	34.02	35.82	35.75 35.93	35.80	35.89	36.00	36.04	36.09	34.89	34.61

Year	*2023*	*2024*
Conversion Factor	33.06	32.74 33.29

2025 Conversion Factor: 32.35

CALCULATING MEDICARE PAYMENTS *(*use the appropriate facility or non-facility PE RVU)*

Medicare payment = [(wRVU x wGPCI) + (PE RVU* x PE GPCI) + (MP RVU x PLI GPCI)] x CF

RBRVS has been criticized for rewarding *effort* and not *outcomes* essentially incentivizing complicated and costly procedures. As a result, physicians often choose specialty careers at the expense of Primary Care.

Although the RBRVS system is mandated by CMS and the data for it appears in the Federal Register, the AMA maintains a copyright of CPT which allows them to charge a license fee to those who wish to associate RVU values with CPT codes. The AMA receives millions of dollars annually in royalties, making them reluctant to allow free distribution of tools and data that might help physicians calculate their fees accurately and fairly.

E/M CODING

THE BASICS

Reasonable and medically necessary are the overarching criteria for payment in addition to the individual requirements of a CPT code. It would not be medically necessary or appropriate to bill a higher level of evaluation and management service when a lower level of service is warranted.

Volume of documentation does not form the basis upon which a specific level of service is billed.

Documentation should support the level of service billed.

Documentation must be legible. The note should be properly dated and contain the reason for the encounter, medical necessity, and a legible signature.

Medicare Consultation Codes. As of January 1, 2010, Medicare no longer recognizes hospital inpatient or office/other outpatient consultation codes. Some private insurers may still recognize these codes.

QHPs (qualified healthcare professionals) in the same group of the same specialty. All providers with the same specialty designation in the same group practice (e.g., reporting services under the same tax identification number) are considered a single entity and must adhere to the global period billing rules. This includes APP's.

New vs. Established patients. A "new" patient is one that has not received professional services in the past 3 years from you or a QHP in the same group of the same specialty.

CPT 99024. As of July 1, 2017, some practitioners are required to report post-operative E/M visits using this code. There is no billable charge attached to this code.

Using disclaimers. Examples include the following: "Due to possible errors in transcription, there may be errors in documentation"; "Due to voice recognition software, sound alike and misspelled words may be contained in the documentation"; and "I am not responsible for errors due to transcription." Providers are responsible for medical record documentation. The provider should verify the information is complete and accurate prior to attaching their signature. *Using disclaimers does not absolve the provider from the medico-legal consequences of inaccurate documentation.*

Copy-pasting and over documentation. The Office of the Inspector General (OIG) in 2014 warned: "Copy-pasting, also known as cloning, enables users to select information from one source and replicate it in another location. When doctors...copy-paste information but fail to update it or ensure accuracy, inaccurate information may enter the patient's medical record and inappropriate charges may be billed to patients and third-party health care payers. Furthermore, inappropriate copy-pasting could facilitate attempts to inflate claims and duplicate or create fraudulent claims."

Non-QHP utilisation for documentation. The CC (chief complaint), Review of Systems (ROS) and the Past, Family, Social History (PFSH) may be recorded by clinical staff or on a form completed by the patient. The QHP must add a notation supplementing or confirming the information recorded by others. The ROS / PFSH obtained during an earlier encounter does not need to be rerecorded if the QHP documents that it was reviewed and updated and notes the date and location of the earlier ROS / PFSH.

"Unremarkable" and "Non-contributory". These terms do not meet appropriate documentation requirements.

Non-patient specific information is unacceptable. Examples include: "if the patient was a smoker, they were advised to stop," or "education was given, if new medications were prescribed." It is difficult and potentially dangerous to design a medical treatment plan in which "one size fits all."

Suspected, rule out, probable, or possible diagnoses or conditions are not coded. Instead, code the sign or symptom.

"Patients over Paperwork" Initiative by CMS.
Input from the AMA Relative Value Scale Update Committee.

General

- Applies to Office / Other Outpatient and Hospital Inpatient Services.
- **Select billing level by Total Time or Medical Decision Making.**
- A **chief complaint** must be documented for every encounter.
- **History and/or Examination need only be "medically appropriate" (determination made by the provider).** This can lead to the unintended consequence of laxity in documentation which can have medico-legal repercussions. **The Joint Commission**, on the other hand, requires that the "medical history and physical examination…should be relevant and include sufficient information necessary to provide care, treatment, and services required to address the patient's condition, planned care, and assessed needs…An H&P must be completed and entered into the medical record for any high-risk procedure, surgical procedure, and any procedure that involves anesthesia services….A dictated H&P that has not been transcribed…is not in compliance with the intent of this requirement."
- Information may be collected by questionnaire or electronic portal – the provider should indicate that this was reviewed.

Selecting Billing Level by Total Time

Face to Face (F2F) encounter is required by one of the providers, but non-F2F time may be included in the total time calculation.
Total time calculation is time spent on the date of service only.
Total time does not apply to 99211 as this service is usually provided by an RN, MA, or office staff. It also does not apply to ER services.

Includes

- EMR review and documentation time.
- Preparing to see the patient (e.g., reviewing tests).
- Obtaining / reviewing separately obtained history.
- Performing a medically appropriate evaluation / examination.
- Counseling / education of patient / family.
- Ordering medications, tests[1], or procedures[1].
- Referring and communicating with other health care providers[1].
- Independent interpretation of results and communicating results to the patient / family / caregiver[1].
- Care coordination[1].

[1]*unless separately reported and billed*

Excludes

- Time spent on a previous or subsequent day.
- Time for activities performed by clinical staff (RNs, MAs, etc.).
- Time that overlaps between NPP and Physician for the purpose of split-shared billing (see below).
- Time spent travelling or general teaching.

TEACHING PHYSICIANS

Primary Care Exception (PCE) Setting: Count only the Teaching Physician or Resident's time, not both.
Non-PCE Setting: Count only the Teaching Physician's time.
In both settings: Do not count time spent in educating the Resident since the institution receives payment for this already.

Selecting Billing Level by Medical Decision Making (MDM)

Requirements for 2 of 3 Elements must be met or exceeded

Element 1: Number & Complexity of Problems Addressed

Includes: Problems evaluated or treated at the encounter.
Excludes:

- Referrals made without evaluation or consideration of treatment.
- Problems that are being managed by another provider without documentation of additional assessment or care coordination by you.
- Comorbidities, unless they are addressed and they impact the other two elements below.

Systemic symptoms: affect 1 or more organ systems and have high risk of morbidity without treatment (e.g., fever as a general symptom in a minor illness does not qualify but fever in another illness with additional patient comorbid factors may qualify).
Final diagnosis alone does not determine complexity or risk.
Chronic illness: illness with an expected duration of ≥ 1 year or until death.
Chronic illnesses not at treatment goal are not considered 'stable' (e.g., poorly controlled blood pressure where the pressures are not changing and patient is asymptomatic is not at the treatment goal of "better control" and therefore not stable).

Element 2: Amount and/or Complexity of Data Reviewed and Analyzed

Eliminates the need for cutting-pasting of results.
Categories include 1) tests, documents, orders, and independent historians, 2) independent interpretation of tests, and 3) discussion of management or test interpretation with external Qualified Healthcare Professional (QHP).
Each unique test, order, or document that is reviewed or analyzed may be counted.
A unique test is defined by the CPT code set. Multiple results of the same unique test (e.g., serial blood glucose values) reviewed during an encounter, count as one unique test. Tests that have overlapping elements are not unique even if they have distinct CPT codes.
Tests ordered that are separately billed by the provider cannot be counted.
An ordered test includes the subsequent review of the result and the review cannot be separately credited on another date of service.
Review of all materials from any unique source counts for a single point.
Independent interpretation of tests requires that the provider reviews the actual raw data (images, tracings, etc.) and not simply the report, and documents their own interpretation which does not need to conform to normal report documentation standards.
External Physician or QHP is an individual who is in a different specialty or subspecialty or who is not in the same group practice, licensed independent practitioners, or a facility.

Element 3: Risk of Complications and/or Morbidity / Mortality of Patient Management

Risk related to patient management is different than the risk of the patient's condition / diagnosis. Risk stratification is based on the usual behavior and thought processes of a physician or other QHP in the same specialty.
In Shared Decision Making, credit is given for discussion of management options, whether that option is selected or declined.
Social Determinants of Health examples include literacy issues, inadequate education, food or housing insecurity, poverty or low income, unemployment, disappearance / illness / death of family member, or child in welfare custody.
'Major' and 'minor' surgery is based on the common meaning of such terms when used by trained clinicians and is not always aligned to surgery global periods (e.g., a Colonoscopy has a 0-day global period yet carries a risk of perforation and would be considered a major procedure).
Monitoring for cytopenia when using an antineoplastic agent qualifies as intensive monitoring for toxicity. Monitoring glucose levels during insulin therapy is monitoring for therapeutic effect and wouldn't qualify.
Elective or Emergency surgery relates to the patient condition. An elective surgery is typically planned in advance. An emergent / urgent surgery is typically performed immediately or after a short period of time required for patient stabilization.
Decision regarding parenteral controlled substances is not solely based on the presence of an order for the parenteral controlled substance.

MEDICAL DECISION MAKING (MDM) BASED CODING

2 of 3 MDM Elements (PROBLEM, DATA, OR RISK) Must Meet or Exceed Requirements for Level Billed.

Documentation Requirement: Chief Complaint and a medically appropriate H&P (as determined by provider).
Medicare patient seen in ER and Admitted by you: use CPT series 9922_ with AI modifier.

	OFFICE / OUTPATIENT			ER	HOSPITAL INPATIENT / OBSERVATION			
	New Patient or Consult Medicare Patient	Established Patient	Consult Non-Medicare Patient		Consult Non-Medicare Patient	Initial Service, Consult Medicare Patient, or Admit for < 8 hrs + DC on same day	Subsequent Service	Admit for 8-24 hrs + DC on same day
CPT Series	9920_	9921_	9924_	9928_	9925_	9922_	9923_	9923_

CPT Code 5th Digit

PROBLEM(S) Addressed & Their Complexity

Self-limited minor.		☐	2, 3[1]	2, 3[1]	1	4
Acute	Stable.	☐	3	3	1	4
	Uncomplicated.	☐	3	3	1	4
	Uncomplicated + requiring hospital level of care.	☐	N/A	3	1	4
	With systemic symptoms.	☐	4	4	2	5
	Complicated injury.	☐	4	4	2	5
Chronic	Stable (at treatment goal).	☐	3, 4[1]	3, 4[1]	1, 2[1]	4, 5[1]
	With exacerbation / progression / treatment side effects.	☐	4	4	2	5
	With severe exacerbation / progression / treatment side effects.	☐	5	5	3	6
New undiagnosed with uncertain prognosis.		☐	4	4	2	5
Acute / Chronic that poses threat to life / bodily function.		☐	5	5	3	6

[1]Select higher level if ≥ 2 problems addressed

DATA Reviewed & Analyzed

Minimal or None.			☐	2	2	1	4
Assessment requiring an independent historian.			☐	3	3	1	4
1 point for: • Notes reviewed from each unique external source. • Each unique test ordered (includes credit for subsequent results review). • Each unique test result reviewed (if not previously ordered). • Assessment requiring an independent historian.	2 points		☐	3	3	1	4
	≥ 3 points	**	☐	4, 5	4, 5	2, 3	5, 6
Independent interpretation of tests performed by another QHP (must include image / tracing interpretation).		**	☐	4, 5	4, 5	2, 3	5, 6
Discussion of management / test interpretation with external QHP / appropriate source.		**	☐	4, 5	4, 5	2, 3	5, 6

**Select higher level if any 2 of these 3 items performed

RISK of Management / Treatment

Minimal or None.			☐	2	2	1	4
Drug Management	Over The Counter drug.		☐	3	3	1	4
	Prescription drug.		☐	4	4	2	5
	Prescription drug requiring intensive monitoring for toxicity.		☐	5	5	3	6
Shared Medical Decision Making Regarding	Surgery	Minor.	☐	3	3	1	4
		Minor with patient / procedure risk factors.	☐	4	4	2	5
		Major Elective.	☐	4	4	2	5
		Major Elective with patient / procedure risk factors.	☐	5	5	3	6
		Major Emergent.	☐	5	5	3	6
	Hospitalization or escalation of hospital level of care.		☐	5	5	3	6
Diagnosis / Treatment significantly limited by SDOH.			☐	4	4	2	5
Extensive discussion re: Diagnosis of Cancer and multiple treatment options (Surgery, Chemo, XRT including risks / benefits).			☐	5	5	3	6
Decision for DNR / de-escalate care due to poor prognosis.			☐	5	5	3	6
Decision regarding parenteral controlled substances.			☐	5	5	3	6

CPT CODE (work RVU):

OFFICE / OUTPATIENT			ER	HOSPITAL INPATIENT / OBSERVATION			
99202 (0.93)	**99212** (0.70)	**99242** (1.08)	**99282** (0.93)	**99252** (1.50)	**99221** (1.63)	**99231** (1.00)	**99234** (2.00)
99203 (1.60)	**99213** (1.30)	**99243** (1.80)	**99283** (1.60)	**99253** (2.00)	**99222** (2.60)	**99232** (1.59)	**99235** (3.24)
99204 (2.60)	**99214** (1.92)	**99244** (2.69)	**99284** (2.74)	**99254** (2.72)	**99223** (3.50)	**99233** (2.40)	**99236** (4.30)
99205 (3.50)	**99215** (2.80)	**99245** (3.75)	**99285** (4.00)	**99255** (3.86)			

TIME BASED CODING

Documentation Requirement:

Chief Complaint and a medically appropriate (as determined by provider) H&P.

Always Time Based Coding: Critical Care and Discharge Services.
Never Time Based Coding: ER Services (refer to MDM Based Coding).

When Split / Sharing: The provider that spends > 50% of the combined total time of both providers would bill.
Documentation PEARL: "I independently spent ___ minutes performing an evaluation and management of this patient, which is > 50% of the total time (___ minutes) of this split / shared service with the APP."

TOTAL TIME: Time spent on the day of the face-to-face (F2F) encounter only. **DO NOT include time spent on other days.**

TOTAL TIME INCLUDES

- Preparing to see the patient (e.g., review of tests).
- Obtaining and / or reviewing separately obtained history.
- Performing a medically appropriate exam / evaluation.
- Counseling and educating the patient / family / caregiver.
- Ordering medications, tests, or procedures.
- Referring and communicating with other healthcare professionals (when not separately reported).
- Documenting clinical information in the Electronic Record.
- Independently interpreting results (not separately reported) and communicating results to the patient / family / caregiver.
- Care coordination.
- Teaching that is specific to the patient and their diagnosis.

TOTAL TIME EXCLUDES

- Services that are reported separately.
- Travel.
- Teaching that is general and not limited to discussion that is required for management.

HOSPITAL SERVICE SPECIAL NOTES

- **Only 1 initial visit per specialty can be billed per admission.**
- **Only 1 subsequent visit per specialty can be billed per day.**
- **When MDM or Total Time spans 2 calendar days, report it as a single service on 1 day.**
- Specialty providers consulted by the ER should bill ER codes (may use modifier 25 on the ER CPT code if the specialty provider also admits the patient and codes for the admission).

OFFICE / OUTPATIENT

	New Patient, or Consultation Medicare Patient		Established Patient		Consultation Non-Medicare Patient	
"Incident To" Service Allowed	NO		YES		NO	
Split / Shared Service Allowed	NO		NO		NO	
TOTAL TIME	Minutes	CPT (wRVU)	Minutes	CPT (wRVU)	Minutes	CPT (wRVU)
	15-29	99202 (0.93)	10-19	99212 (0.70)	20-29	99242 (1.08)
	30-44	99203 (1.60)	20-29	99213 (1.30)	30-39	99243 (1.80)
	45-59	99204 (2.60)	30-39	99214 (1.92)	40-54	99244 (2.69)
	60-74	99205 (3.50)	40-54	99215 (2.80)	55-69	99245 (3.75)
Prolonged Services	*99417 (0.61) (each additional full 15 mins)*					
MD not required (Staff service only)			*99211 (0.18)*			

HOSPITAL INPATIENT / OBSERVATION

	Initial Service, Consultation Medicare Patient, or Admit for < 8 hours + D/C same day		Subsequent Service		Admit for 8 to 24 hours + D/C same day		Consultation Non-Medicare Patient	
Split / Shared Service Allowed	YES		YES		YES		NO	
TOTAL TIME	Minutes	CPT (wRVU)	Minutes	CPT (wRVU)	Minutes	CPT (wRVU)	Minutes	CPT (wRVU)
	40-54	99221 (1.63)	25-34	99231 (1.00)	45-69	99234 (2.00)	34-44	99252 (1.50)
							45-59	99253 (2.00)
	55-74	99222 (2.60)	35-49	99232 (1.59)	70-84	99235 (3.24)	60-79	99254 (2.72)
	75-89	99223 (3.50)	50-64	99233 (2.40)	85-99	99236 (4.30)	80-94	99255 (3.86)
Prolonged Services	*99418 (0.81) (each add'l full 15 mins)*							

CRITICAL CARE / DISCHARGE

	CRITICAL CARE		DISCHARGE	
Split / Shared Service Allowed	YES		YES	
ALWAYS TIME BASED	Minutes	CPT (wRVU)	Minutes	CPT (wRVU)
	< 30	9922__ or 9923__	≤ 30	99238 (0.70)
	30-74	99291 (4.50)	> 30	99239 (1.30)
	Each add'l 30 min	99292 (2.25)		
Post-op Critical Care Unrelated to Surgical Procedure	*Use Modifier FT*			

ER

	ER
Split / Shared Service Allowed	YES
NEVER TIME BASED (REFER TO MDM BASED CODING)	CPT (wRVU)
	99282 (0.93)
	99283 (1.60)
	99284 (2.74)
	99285 (4.00)
MD not required (Staff service only)	*99281 (0.48)*

CONSULTATIONS

On January 1, 2010, Medicare eliminated payment for all CPT consultation codes (99241 to 99245 and 99251 to 99255).

CONSULTATION: a request for advice or opinion regarding evaluation or management of a specific problem.

- Consults may be requested by persons other than physicians (e.g., physician assistants, nurse practitioners, chiropractors, physical therapists, psychologists, social workers, lawyers or insurance carriers).
- With the consulting physician's advice as a guide, the requestor intends to continue to treat the patient.
- Consultations cannot be requested by the patient or family members.

TRANSFER OF CARE / REFERRAL:

- **Occurs "when a physician requests that another physician take over the responsibility for managing the patient's complete care for the condition and does not expect to continue treating or caring for the patient for that condition."** For example, a patient who does not have a primary care physician seeks care at an urgent care facility and is sent to a primary care physician to establish ongoing care. This is not a consultation. A statement such as "Thank you for referring this patient to me for left inguinal hernia repair," indicates that transfer of care occurred at the time the referral was made.
- This also applies when a patient is referred from the ER.
- Should the requesting physician transfer the care of this patient to the consultant after the initial consult/initiation of care, return patient visits would be coded as appropriate subsequent inpatient or outpatient care.

DOCUMENTATION REQUIREMENTS:

- **Request for consultation by the requesting physician.** A verbal consultation request alone does not meet this requirement. Must include how the consultant was contacted (e.g., phone, fax, or letter). Likewise, the consultant should document that a consultation was requested, by whom and why.
- **Reason for the consultation.**
- **Report of the consultation service, findings, and recommendations or planned follow-up.** The report is not a thank you note to the requesting physician for referring the patient, nor is it a courtesy copy of the history and physical. Rather, the report provides instruction to allow the requesting physician to continue treating the patient.

SPECIAL SITUATIONS:

- **Inpatient settings:** You may bill an inpatient consultation code provided in the hospital only once per admission. If you are consulted again during the admission, you should report a subsequent hospital service code.
- **Outpatient settings:** The consultant can use an initial office consultation code. If the consultant initiates follow-up services in the office or other outpatient facility, the follow-up services should be reported using the office established patient services codes.
- **Consultations mandated by third-party payers** (e.g., a mandatory second opinion): Should be reported with modifier 32. Medicare does not recognize modifier 32 for payment.
- **Preoperative clearance:** A surgeon may request preoperative clearance from the patient's primary care physician. For example, do the comorbid conditions of this patient require any special considerations? Can this patient safely undergo this procedure?

  Use the appropriate consultation code as well as diagnosis codes that indicate the necessity of the consultation (e.g., V72.81 for preoperative cardiovascular exam, V72.82 for a preoperative respiratory exam, V72.83 for another specified preoperative exam or V72.84 for an unspecified preoperative exam) and secondary codes to indicate the condition for which surgery is intended and any diagnoses that arise during your consultation. If after the initial consultation, the consultant assumes care for a portion of the patient's condition during the postoperative period, then consultation codes should not be used on subsequent visits.
- **Postoperative evaluation** that is performed at the request of the surgeon can be billed using a consultation code as long as all consultation criteria are documented and a preoperative consultation was not already performed. You cannot bill a consultation if you are asked simply to manage an aspect of the patient's condition during the postop period, because the surgeon is not asking for your opinion or advice in treating the patient. Instead, this service would constitute concurrent care.
- **Shared/Split service:** When a qualified nonphysician practitioner (NPP) and a physician each provide a portion of the consultation services. Consultations cannot be billed as shared/split services.
- **Consults can include treatment as long as the visit meets all consultation criteria and no transfer of care occurs.** If the consultant initiates treatment at the time of the consult, he may add a statement like, "I performed excisional biopsy while she was here for consultation, and am awaiting the pending pathology report."
- **Group or specialty physicians can request consults**: Same-specialty or same-practice consultations are allowed "when the consulting physician has expertise in a specific medical area beyond the requesting professional's knowledge."

  "A consultation service *shall not* be reported on *every* patient as a routine practice between physicians within a group practice setting" because of the tendency for abuse. The requesting physician should clarify in the documentation that the same-specialty / practice consultant truly has a skill set the requester does not have.

(see the next page for Scenarios for clarification)

Scenario 1: A general surgeon is consulted by a patient's internist for evaluation of a breast mass. The surgeon documents the request for the consult from the requesting physician, history, exam and medical decision making, and any diagnostic or therapeutic procedures ordered or performed in evaluating the breast mass. The surgeon determines that a FNA biopsy is necessary to further evaluate the mass. He documents communication to the patient's internist of his findings of a diagnosis of fibrocystic breast disease which does not warrant further surgical care / intervention at this time. The patient returns to her internist for follow-up care. The surgeon can bill for the initial office consultation, as well as the biopsy performed on the same day.

Scenario 2: A general surgeon is consulted by a patient's internist for evaluation of a breast mass that is clinically suspicious by Mammogram. The surgeon determines that further surgery is needed to remove the mass or breast and assumes care for this specific problem. The consulting physician documents communication of his findings to the internist at which time the internist transfers the care of the patient over to the surgeon for further surgical care / intervention for the breast mass. The surgeon would not bill a consultation code. He would bill an office new / established patient service code.

Scenario 3: A pulmonologist sees a patient at the primary-care physician's (PCP) request. The consultation request specifies, "Patient wheezing indicates that she may suffer from asthma. Please provide additional workup and your opinion on treatment options." This service has a request and reason, and the PCP clarifies his wishes to continue to treat the patient for the possible asthma. If the pulmonologist responds with a written report outlining a care plan and possible treatment options, he has met all consultation requirements and can bill a consultation code.

Scenario 4: An ED physician treats a patient for a sprained ankle by applying ACE wrap. The ED physician discharges the patient and advises him to visit an orthopedic clinic for follow-up. In this case, the orthopedist would not bill a consultation code because the ED physician isn't really seeking the orthopedist's advice or opinion. This scenario indicates a transfer of care and the orthopedist would bill an office new / established patient service code.

Scenario 5: A patient visits his PCP with chest pains consistent with unstable angina. The PCP requests a consultation from a cardiologist to evaluate the patient and to provide treatment recommendations. The cardiologist performs a diagnostic heart cath, which showed minimal disease, writes a prescription for the patient, and prepares a letter with findings and recommendations for ongoing care. Even though the cardiologist initiated the care, the service meets all the consultation requirements and may be reported as such.

Scenario 6: An ENT specialist sees a patient who complains of left-side-only hearing loss. He suspects an acoustic neuroma due to the single-sided nature of the problem, and requests a consultation with a neuro-otologist in the same practice. As long as the service meets all the consult requirements (request, reason, and report), the neuro-otologist may report the service with the appropriate office consultation code.

CRITICAL CARE

Definition

Critical care is the direct delivery of medical care for a critically ill or critically injured patient. A critical illness or injury acutely impairs one or more vital organ systems such that there is a high probability of imminent or life-threatening deterioration in the patient's condition (e.g., CNS failure, circulatory failure, shock, renal / hepatic / metabolic / and/or respiratory failure, etc.). Usually involves high complexity decision making to assess, manipulate, and support vital system functions to treat single or multiple vital organ system failure and/or to prevent further life-threatening deterioration of the patient's condition. Typically includes interpretation of multiple physiologic parameters and/or application of advanced technologies.

The illness or injury and the treatment being provided meet the above requirements.

While critical care is usually given in the ICU or ER, any location qualifies as long as this care meets the critical care definition.

New in 2022, Critical care services can be shared/split services.

Medical Necessity

Critical care services must be *reasonable and medically necessary* and must encompass both:

- **the treatment of "vital organ failure", and**
- **the "prevention of further life-threatening deterioration in the patient's condition."**

Therefore, delivering critical care in a moment of crisis, or upon being called to the patient's bedside emergently, is not the only requirement for providing critical care service. **Providing care to a critically ill patient does not automatically qualify as a critical care service just because the patient is critically ill.**

The following are not considered critical care services:

- Daily management of a patient on chronic ventilator therapy or management of dialysis for a patient with ESRF who is in the ICU, unless the critical care is separately identifiable from the chronic long-term management of the ventilator dependence or dialysis dependence.
- Services provided to a patient admitted to an ICU a) because no other hospital beds were available, or b) because hospital rules require certain treatments (e.g., Insulin infusion) to be administered in the ICU
- Services provided to a patient by an assigned provider to an ICU (e.g., Hospitalist, Intensivist, etc.) simply because the patient is in the ICU.

Time and Full Attention

Documentation must include total time (the time actually spent on evaluating, managing, and providing care). The time may be continuous or aggregated intermittent time. Only one provider may bill for the critical care service during any one single period of time even if more than one physician is providing care during that time. **During this time, you cannot provide services to any other patient and must devote your *full* attention to this particular critically ill patient. You may not use time spent teaching and cannot include a resident's time.**

Special Situations

- The following are bundled in the critical care services and should not be billed separately:
  - interpretation of cardiac output measurements, professional component of chest x-rays, blood draw for specimen, blood gases and information data stored in computers (EKG, etc.), gastric intubation, pulse oximetry, temporary transcutaneous pacing, ventilator management, vascular access procedures).
  - *routine daily updates to family members* and/or surrogates are bundled with the critical care service and may be counted towards the time criteria if it is required to obtain a history or discuss treatment options with family in cases where:
    - the patient is unable or incompetent to give a history or make treatment decisions, and
    - the discussion is necessary for determining treatment decisions.

    Documentation must clearly show that these requirements have been met. (e.g., "no other source was available to obtain a history" or "because the patient was rapidly deteriorating, I needed to immediately discuss treatment options with the family.")
- Critical care services on the day of a global surgical procedure may be billed separately with modifier 25 or FT only if it is a "significant, separately identifiable service above and beyond the usual pre- and post- operative care associated with the procedure".
- *Endotracheal intubation, Swan-Ganz catheter insertion, and CPR* are not bundled with the critical care codes and may be billed separately with modifier 25. The time performing the pre-, intra-, and post- procedure work should be excluded from the determination of the time spent providing the critical care service.
- Critical care services for *trauma and burn cases* during the pre- and post- operative portions of a 90-day global procedure may be paid if:
  - the patient is critically ill and requires the full attention of the physician, and
  - the critical care is unrelated to the specific anatomic injury or general surgical procedure performed.

  Documentation must clearly show that the requirements have been met (e.g., "this critical care service is unrelated to the procedure.")

Documentation Pearl: "I have personally spent total time of ____ minutes evaluating, managing, and providing care for this patient. During this time, my attention was devoted exclusively to this patient and does not include time spent on critical care bundled services. This patient has a critical illness that acutely impairs one or more vital organ systems and there is a high probability of imminent or life-threatening deterioration in the patient's condition. My supporting documentation is as follows: …"

USING NPPs IN YOUR PRACTICE

NPPs (non-Physician Practitioners): Nurse Practitioners (NPs), Physician Assistants (PAs), Clinical Nurse Specialists (CNSs), and Certified Nurse Midwives (CNMs).

Applies to Medicare. Private contractors may have different interpretations of these rules.

- **All E/M services must be "reasonable and necessary".**
- **The E/M level of care should be supported by the documentation.**
- **Services performed by an NPP must be within the NPP's scope of practice.**

Physicians billing 'incident to' and 'shared / split' services are paid at 100% of the Medicare Physician Fee Schedule.
NPPs billing are paid at 85% of the physician fee schedule.

PLACE OF SERVICE

Office / Clinic	use Incident To service billing
Hospital (Inpatient / Outpatient / Observation / Discharge / Critical Care / ER)	use Shared / Split service billing

"INCIDENT TO" SERVICE

- Physician must personally perform the initial E/M service and remain actively involved in the course of treatment. Physician would bill for this initial service. 'Incident to' services cannot be rendered on the patient's first visit or if a change to the plan of care occurs. If the patient has a new or worsening complaint, the physician must conduct an E/M service for that complaint and must establish the diagnosis and update the plan of care and would bill for those services.
- Physician may bill 'incident to' for subsequent established patient visits if the following criteria is met:
  - ✓ NPP provides services to an existing patient with a physician-established plan of care that are an integral, although incidental, part of the physician's professional service.
  - ✓ NPP sees the patient for the pre-determined plan of care.
  - ✓ Physician must be present in the office suite and immediately available to provide assistance and direction.
  - ✓ NPP must be directly employed by the physician, physician group, or entity that employs the physician.
- NPP would bill if:
  - ✓ NPP performs the initial E/M service on a new patient.
  - ✓ NPP alone sees an established patient with a new problem.
  - ✓ Physician is not present in the office suite.

SUMMARY	
New Patient Initial Visit	• If you wish to use "incident to" services for future visits, the Physician must personally perform the initial E/M service, determine a plan of care, and remain actively involved in the course of treatment. This initial E/M service would be billed under the Physician. • If you do not wish to use "incident to" services, the NPP can perform the initial E/M service and this would be billed under the NPP. All subsequent services provided by the NPP would also be billed under the NPP. The Physician would not be able to bill for any services provided by the NPP.
Established Patient Subsequent Visit (No change in the plan of care, No new or worsening complaints)	• NPP can see the patient and document a service and the Physician may bill for the service.
Established Patient Subsequent Visit (Requires a change in the plan of care or has a new or worsening complaint)	• "Incident to" services cannot be rendered. For the Physician to bill, he/she must conduct the E/M service and must establish the diagnosis and update the plan of care. • If you do not wish to use "incident to" services, the NPP can provide this E/M service and it would be billed under the NPP.

(Shared/Split visit on next page ...)

"SHARED/SPLIT" SERVICE

Occurs when both a physician and a qualified NPP each perform a portion of the E/M visit.
The work of the physician and the NPP are "combined" into a single E/M service.

Excludes: Procedures (at any Place of Service) and Consultations.

- Physician service and NPP service may occur jointly or at independent times throughout the day as long as they occur on the same calendar day.
- A face-to-face encounter by only one of the providers is required although both may provide it. The physician is not mandated to provide a face-to-face encounter.
- Modifier FS should be appended to the charge to signify that the service was a shared/split service.

DETERMINE WHETHER YOU WILL BE BILLING BY SUBSTANTIVE PORTION OR TOTAL TIME

Critical Care Service (time-based billing)	Non-Critical Care Service (Hospital Inpatient / Observation, ER, etc.)
Use Total Time option only (See page 23 for other requirements)	**Use Substantive portion option or Total Time option**

Option 1: Substantive portion method

For the physician to bill for the shared/split service: *(if all these are not met, NPP would bill for the service)*

- ✓ Physician must perform a F2F service and make/approve the medical decision making for the problems addressed, thereby taking responsibility for the plan's inherent risk of complications/morbidity/mortality.
  - If the physician's participation is only reviewing the patient's medical record, the service should be billed by the NPP.
  - It is not sufficient for physician to document "seen and agree" or simply countersign the NPP's note.
- ✓ Physician must date and legibly sign the medical record (or have an electronic signature in the EMR).
- ✓ The physician and NPP should each personally document his/her portion of the E/M shared/split service.

Option 2: Total Time method

The provider that performs >50% of the combined total time of the service would bill for the service.

- ✓ Both providers must document their individual time spent evaluating and managing the patient. The documentation should clearly identify what each provider did during that time.
- ✓ Total time may be contiguous or aggregated intermittent time.

ACCEPTABLE PHYSICIAN DOCUMENTATION

"I personally saw and examined the patient and discussed the management with the NPP. I reviewed the NPP note and have made corrections as follows: *[insert here]*. I performed the following evaluation and management services personally which includes addressing problems and formulating medical decision making: *[insert here]*."

UNACCEPTABLE PHYSICIAN DOCUMENTATION

Such documentation is not acceptable as it is not possible to determine whether the Physician was present, evaluated the patient, and/or had any involvement in the plan of care.

- Any of the following: "Agree with above," "Rounded, Reviewed, Agree," "Discussed with NPP. Agree," "Seen and agree," "As above," "Patient seen," or "Patient seen and evaluated," followed by a legible countersignature.
- A legible countersignature alone.
- "Dr. X saw the patient with me and agrees with my plan." The NPP cannot document for the Physician.

GLOBAL PERIOD

<table>
<tr><th>GLOBAL PERIOD</th><th>NOTES</th><th colspan="2">BILLABLE EXCEPTIONS TO THE GLOBAL PERIOD</th></tr>
<tr><td>0-Day
(Endoscopy, anterior abdominal wall hernia repairs, and some minor procedures)</td><td>• No pre-operative or post-operative period.</td><td rowspan="2">Use modifier 25 when coding for a significant, separately identifiable E/M service on the same day as a minor surgery or Endoscopy.</td><td rowspan="3">• Visits unrelated to the diagnosis for which the surgical procedure is performed (use modifier 24).
• Treatment for the underlying condition or an added course of treatment which is not part of normal recovery from surgery.
• Clearly distinct surgical procedures that occur during the post-operative period which are not re-operations or treatment for complications. A new global period begins with the subsequent procedure (use modifier 79).
• Treatment for complications <u>requiring</u> return to the operating room (use modifier 78).
• Staged procedures (use modifier 58).
• Critical care services unrelated to the surgery where a seriously injured or burned patient is critically ill and requires constant attendance of the physician (use modifier 25 or FT).</td></tr>
<tr><td>10-Day
(other minor procedures)</td><td>• No pre-operative period.
• Total global period is 11 days. The day of the surgery is day 0 and then 10 subsequent days.</td></tr>
<tr><td>90-Day
(major procedures)</td><td>• One day pre-operative included.
• Total global period is 92 days. Count 1 day before the surgery, the day of surgery, and the 90 subsequent days.</td><td>Use modifier 57 when coding for the initial E/M service when the decision to perform major surgery is made.</td></tr>
</table>

Operating Room: a surgical operating room, cardiac catheterization suite, or an endoscopy suite. It does not include the patient's room, minor treatment room, recovery room, or ICU (unless the patient's condition was so critical there would be insufficient time for transportation to an OR).

SERVICES INCLUDED IN THE GLOBAL SURGERY PACKAGE (may not be billed separately)

- Pre-op visits **after** the initial decision to perform surgery has already been made.
- Intra-op services that are normally a usual and necessary part of a surgical procedure (e.g. lysis of adhesions during a major abdominal surgery, laparoscopy that determines that the surgery needs to be converted to an open procedure, or umbilical hernia repair during an abdominal surgery that requires a midline incision).
- Services during the post-op period for:
  - Follow-up visits related to surgical recovery.
  - Treatment for complications <u>not</u> requiring return to the operating room.
  - Post-op pain management by the surgeon.
  - Supplies, except for those identified as exclusions.
  - Miscellaneous services (dressing changes, local incision care, removal of sutures / staples / lines / wires / tubes / drains, urinary catheter insertion / irrigation / removal, peripheral IV line care, nasogastric / rectal tubes, and tracheostomy tube change / removal).

RELATED, STAGED, OR UNRELATED SERVICES

The reason for the original surgery and for the subsequent procedure must be considered.

Related (reimbursement is already included in the global surgery fee for the original surgery)
- Services treating complications from the original surgery.
- Procedures to treat or assist with expected developments in the healing process.
- Services associated with returning the patient to the appropriate post-procedure state.
- Services on the operative site or contiguous structures when the subsequent procedure would not have been needed if the original surgery had never been performed.

Unrelated (reimbursement may be paid separately)
- Procedures to treat the same or similar problems in the contralateral, non-operative organ, extremity, or joint.
- Services on a different body organ or unrelated operative site (when the subsequent procedure would have been needed even if the original surgery had never been performed).

Staged (reimbursement may be paid separately)
When the subsequent procedure is:
- planned or anticipated and being performed for the same diagnosis as the original surgery.
- more extensive than the first because the desired outcome was not accomplished.
- performed to "finish" what was started with the original surgery.
- being done to facilitate therapy.

MODIFIERS FOR E/M SERVICES	
24	**Unrelated E/M service by the same physician during a postoperative period.** An E/M service that was performed during a postoperative period for a reason(s) unrelated to the original procedure.
25	**Significant, separately identifiable E/M service by the same physician on the same day of the procedure or other service.** In certain instances, the patient's condition may require a significant, separately identifiable E/M service above and beyond the other service provided or beyond the usual preoperative and postoperative care associated with the procedure that was performed. The E/M service may be prompted by the symptom or condition for which the procedure and/or service was provided. As such, different diagnosis is not required for reporting of E/M services on the same date. **This modifier is not used to report an E/M service that results in a decision to perform surgery - see modifier 57.**
26	**Professional component.** Applies to certain procedures that have a combination of a professional component and technical component and are performed in an inpatient or outpatient setting. Where the physician provides the professional component only. The facility may be reimbursed for the technical component.
32	**Mandated services.** Services related to mandated consultation and/or related services (e.g., third party payer, governmental, legislative or regulatory requirement).
55	**Postoperative management only.** When one physician performs the postoperative care and another physician has performed the surgical procedure.

GC	**Teaching physician.** When a service has been performed in part by a resident under the direction of a teaching physician
GE	When a service has been performed by a resident without the presence of a teaching physician under the primary care exception

FS	Shared/split service modifier.
FT	Critical care service performed by surgeon / same specialty during a global period

APPENDIX A: SHETH'S EMR BEST PRACTICES

EMR's have many benefits from creating reminders for preventative care and chronic disease management to global access of the medical record chart from any location. And they are legible! Unfortunately, EMR's are also a double-edged sword. EMR's ***will*** slow you down. They are essentially built for data collection and not for clinical efficiency. In an effort to mitigate this, most practitioners unscrupulously use functions such as "copy-and-paste" and rarely use due diligence in checking the accuracy of the information prior to signing the chart. Practitioners are faced with sitting in front of computers for long periods of time, and the **art** of obtaining and documenting a good History and Physical Exam is waning. The integrity of the patient's EMR can be maintained only if all the stakeholders (patient and providers) actively curate it. Parts of the **21st Century Cures Act** (from The Office of the National Coordinator for Health Information Technology) focus on patient access to healthcare records and the prevention of information blocking. It went into effect November 1, 2020 and provides transparency to patients allowing them to participate in their own healthcare.

1. **Utilize the functionality of the EMR's patient History database.** Most physicians do not know where to input a patient's medical / surgical history. Updating the patient History database is tedious. It is easier to simply dictate the history. The drawback to dictating is that the information resides solely in your note and will not be available for future healthcare providers to easily access. Easier for you means harder for others. A better approach is to enter the information into the database fields of the medical / surgical history that is attached to the patient's chart. This will then be carried forward for all healthcare providers to easily access. If everyone does their part, tedious as it is, everyone benefits, including the patient.

2. **Too many cooks ruin the pot.** Be obsessive-compulsive and check the History database each time you see the patient. *Do not assume that the information is accurate.*

   It is not uncommon for a patient's PMH to show the same diagnosis multiple times. "Diabetes", "Diabetes mellitus", and "Diabetes, type 2" – all on the same patient and all inserted by different providers. This exposes the fact that the physician did not review the PMH.

   Follow-up visits can be problematic. Recheck the information in the EMR database for changes. Data may have been deleted or changed and contain incorrect information. I had performed an EGD on a patient and had listed "Gastritis by endoscopy...Dr. Sheth" in the PMH. That patient returned to me a few months later and this information had been deleted without my knowledge and had to be reinserted.

3. **The worst documented section is the Social History.** When possible, document the patient's Occupation and use of Tobacco, Alcohol, or Recreational Drugs. The patient will often say "no" to the question "do you smoke?" However, when followed with the question "have you ever smoked and when did you quit?" the patient may say "last night because I knew I was going to be admitted."

4. **Avoid the following phrases:**

   a. "The PMH/PSH, Meds, Allergies, SH, and FH were reviewed with the patient and updated as necessary". If you use this phrase, make sure you actually did this. A propagated error will easily disprove the above attestation.

   b. "10 systems were reviewed and pertinent positives and negatives listed and all other systems are negative." There is no way to determine which 10 systems were reviewed; therefore, credit cannot be given for the ROS. Instead, you should either list out which 10 systems you have reviewed, or if you reviewed all systems, use the terminology "all 14 systems were reviewed and pertinent positives and negatives are listed".

5. **For cancer diagnoses, add details in the comments section.**

   Example: "Breast cancer: diagnosed 03/2018, infiltrating ductal with DCIS, right breast, UOQ, T2 N0 M0 (Stage 1), ER+, PR+, Her2neu unamplified, s/p L+SLNB, adjuvant Tamoxifen and XRT, SURGEON: Dr. Smith, ONCOLOGIST: Dr. James" is much better than simply "Breast cancer".

6. **Don't use *"CUT-PASTE and SIGN"*.** It can lead to error propagation. Malpractice attorneys, on the other hand, are fond of "copy-and-paste" because they can easily discredit you based on poor documentation. Best practice is to use ***"CUT-PASTE-REVIEW-UPDATE...then SIGN"***. The Office of the Inspector General (OIG) in 2014 warned: "Copy-pasting, also known as cloning, enables users to select information from one source and replicate it in another location. When doctors ... copy-paste information but fail to update it or ensure accuracy, inaccurate information may enter the patient's medical record and inappropriate charges may be billed to patients and third-party health care payers. Furthermore, inappropriate copy-pasting could facilitate attempts to inflate claims and duplicate or create fraudulent claims."

Example: A male patient had "hysterectomy" listed in the PSH...on multiple practitioner notes! It was clear that each practitioner was simply copying the information from the previous note.

7. **APSO notes** (Assessment-Plan-Subjective-Objective) emerged due to electronic SOAP notes being of excessive length, making it difficult to find the actual Assessment and Plan. This is a result of the improper practice of dot-phrase pasting of lengthy labs and full X-ray reports as well as previous daily assessments. Well written SOAP notes on the other hand are succinct, thoughtful, and facilitate patient care (see excerpt below).

8. **Use Physical Exam templates cautiously.** If the template has pre-filled normal findings, remember to update it with any abnormal findings. I have often seen "Extremities: no deformities" on patients with amputations or in the most egregious case, a patient with congenital syndactyly.

9. **Strategically updating PMH / PSH will create a more robust history database.**

    a. **New diagnoses at admission or discharge.** If a patient was admitted after an MVA and had suffered rib fractures and pneumothorax managed by a chest tube, small subdural hemorrhage managed without surgery, and skin laceration of the knee that was sutured, then add MVA to the PMH along with the date of injury and under the comments, insert all the injuries.

    b. **Incidental diagnoses contained in radiologic test results.** Some examples of incidental findings include "atherosclerotic aorto-iliac disease," "diverticulosis," and "coronary calcifications." Adding these incidental findings to the PMH with a comment that they were identified on CT scan will enrich the patient's medical history with potential co-morbidities.

    c. **When surgical procedures are performed.** Add the diagnosis found during the surgical procedure in the PMH. Also include the date of the procedure and the proceduralist name in the comments section.

10. **Avoid ambiguous diagnoses and surgical procedures.** Diagnoses such as "Disease of the thyroid gland" or "Hernia" and surgical procedures like "Hernia repair" are essentially meaningless. Documenting "Hypothyroidism," "Graves' Disease," "Inguinal hernia," or "Right inguinal hernia repair – Robotic laparoscopic – with mesh" is more helpful.

11. **Avoid using disclaimers.** Examples include: "Due to possible errors in transcription, there may be errors in documentation"; "Due to voice recognition software, sound alike and misspelled words may be contained in the documentation"; and "I am not responsible for errors due to transcription." **Providers are responsible for medical record documentation.** The provider should verify the information is complete and accurate prior to attaching their signature. *Using disclaimers does not absolve the provider from the medico-legal consequences of inaccurate documentation.*

12. **Take extra time to make your EMR templates.** The initial effort will pay off in the long run. When I used an EMR for the first time, I was informed that Microsoft Word templates would easily import. In reality, the EMR proprietary word processor stripped off all the customizations in my Microsoft Word templates. I was only able to maintain efficiency by designing my templates as tables and then importing them into the EMR.

13. **Work with your vendor to correct any limitations to the EMR that affect your efficiency.** Most vendors will say "it can't be done easily", "we can put in a ticket", or "we will consider it for the next major update". Do not settle for this. Request that changes be made expeditiously.

14. **A final word. Be extra vigilant in documenting well. "If it is not documented, you didn't do it."**

> An increasing problem encountered with the electronic record is the "cut and paste" phenomena: documentation from one day is cut and pasted to the next rather than constructed anew, and a deluge of laboratory and radiologic information is pasted into daily progress notes and discharge summaries. **These are both abuses of the electronic format that are to be condemned.** Neither requires that the cutter-paster has actually read the material, given it any thought, or reflected upon the whole of the information to form a new and evolving clinical assessment and management plan.
>
> Each daily note should be constructed in its entirety each day, with appropriate references to existing records. The physical findings must be ascertained and recorded daily as they change and evolve. Test results should be succinct summaries of key radiographic findings and the few key chemistry and microbiologic reports used today to make diagnoses or change the management plan. **All the detailed radiologic and laboratory information is readily available to everyone reading the note in another part of the record and it need not be duplicated.**
>
> Electronic records are a boon to patient care when generated and used correctly. Unfortunately, they also facilitate sloppy, expedient but unprofessional and potentially dangerous documentation practices that discourage thought and reflection and perpetuate misstatements, erroneous conclusions and frank errors.
>
> *--- DeGowin's Diagnostic Exam, 9th Edition*

ABOUT ME

Piyush N. Sheth, MD, FACS, DABS, CGSC*

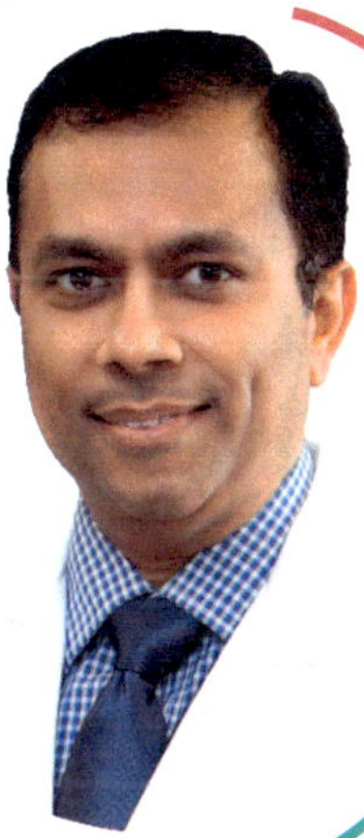

Work Experience

Advanced Surgical Professionals – Solo General Surgery Practice, 1996-2006

Richland Surgical Associates – Single Specialty General Surgery Group, 2006-2015

Employed General Surgeon, 2015-current

Achievements

Outstanding Young Physician by Ohio Medicine, 1998

Outstanding Specialty Medicine Physician Award by Ohio University Heritage College of Osteopathic Medicine, 2017, 2022

Education

Northwestern University, BA degree, 1986

Loyola University Stritch School of Medicine, MD degree, 1990

Loyola University Medical Center, PGY1

Medical College of Ohio, PGY2 to PGY5

Published Books

General Surgery, Trauma, and Vascular Surgery – Medical Student and Resident Manual

Coding Solutions – General Surgery

Coding Solutions – Evaluation and Management Services

Starting Medical Practice

Certifications

Fellow of the American College of Surgeons

Diplomate of the American Board of Surgery

AAPC Certified General Surgery Coder, 2019, 2021

Contact Info

Shethpn.CodingSolutions@gmail.com

Made in United States
Cleveland, OH
06 November 2026

47771493R00017